FROZEN SHOULDER:

SURVIVAL GUIDE

A Nurse's Journey of Discovery,
Diagnosis, and Holistic Healing

Patti Gilliano-McClung, MSN RN

BALBOA.PRESS
A DIVISION OF HAY HOUSE

Balboa Press books may be ordered through booksellers or by contacting:

Balboa Press
A Division of Hay House
1663 Liberty Drive
Bloomington, IN 47403
www.balboapress.com
1 (877) 407-4847

Because of the dynamic nature of the Internet, any web addresses or links contained in this book may have changed since publication and may no longer be valid. The views expressed in this work are solely those of the author and do not necessarily reflect the views of the publisher, and the publisher hereby disclaims any responsibility for them.

The author of this book does not dispense medical advice or prescribe the use of any technique as a form of treatment for physical, emotional, or medical problems without the advice of a physician, either directly or indirectly. The intent of the author is only to offer information of a general nature to help you in your quest for emotional and spiritual well-being. In the event you use any of the information in this book for yourself, which is your constitutional right, the author and the publisher assume no responsibility for your actions.

Any people depicted in stock imagery provided by Getty Images are models, and such images are being used for illustrative purposes only.
Certain stock imagery © Getty Images.

Print information available on the last page.

ISBN: 978-1-9822-5158-1 (sc)
ISBN: 978-1-9822-5160-4 (hc)
ISBN: 978-1-9822-5159-8 (e)

Library of Congress Control Number: 2020913309

Balboa Press rev. date: 07/24/2020

CONTENTS

Welcome to my world, my fellow frozen shoulder friend. Prior to the onset of my first diagnosis of frozen shoulder, I was a nurse, a mom, and an active athlete of sorts. The first thing to know, as an advanced practice nurse of nearly 30 years, I do not always subscribe to the typical medical model. I have seen much in healthcare and dealt with a myriad of issues in treating and healing my family that I am convinced there are many schools of thought, and I prescribe to a holistic approach wherever possible. That said, there are options for treatment I will share so you can have ideas to know what is out there so you can make an informed choice. Do your homework and feel comfortable with your practitioner. My clinical work, and years of professional practice and fitness training and certifications were an advantage to manage my own path of treatment options and fitness therapy. Those of you who find yourself with a diagnosis of frozen shoulder (FS) also known as adhesive capsulitis, make sure you consider not just options, but complications or effects of whatever treatment chosen. I always say, a quick fix is not the permanent solution either. If your FS came on without warning, and sort of crept upon you, then it is what we call, "idiopathic." It happened for some unknown or underlying not yet detectable reason. Later in this book, we will also note a few other ways FS can develop, but for now we will go with no known reason.

It started one morning, as I felt a twinge in my right scapula, I began to think something just was not right. I brushed it off and continued about my day. I had a new wellness center to manage and planned to do a cross-fit class in the evening. The kids had after school activities, and I did not have time for a little soreness. I went on about my day. Later that week, the pain in my shoulder grew worse. As the days pushed on, and I had this stiffness and soreness that would not go away, I began to think, what is going on with my shoulder? The initial discomfort felt like the joint was thick, like something was swollen and irritated inside. I could not imagine what I had done to it. The last thing I remembered, there was a tightness in my scapula as I had taken off my workout top and thought I must have pulled something in my shoulder.

Being athletic my entire life, I consider myself an exercise enthusiast. Many years I was involved in fitness training and athletic events, so I know the feeling of overworking a body part and when to slow down. I have always been active, and running around with three boys, even coaching their soccer teams for a while. Finding myself with restricted movement, was an odd feeling, as I had always been healthy with never a major injury.

Months prior, I had started down the road of cross-fit classes in between launching my own business. Now, with limited range of motion, work and exercise, was not going to be easy. I contemplated just taking a week or so to rest the shoulder to give it time to heal and recover, but even with a few days of babying it, the pain never subsided. I tried a few NSAIDS (non-steroidal anti-inflammatories), with a little success. However, the thickness inside my shoulder just felt odd. It almost felt like a sock balled up inside and was just in the wrong place, but I could not get that feeling to go away for anything.

WORKING THROUGH IT

Initially, I still could not figure out if this shoulder or scapula issue was really an injury or what it could be, because there was not a moment of trauma or insult to my body. I did not fall, or lift a heavy weight, or anything like it, so I really had no idea what happened to my body. I have always leaned on the holistic approach, so thinking I needed to soothe myself, I went for a visit to the chiropractor and then to a massage. Both were helpful, and yet the pain never went away. It just stabbed back in the scapula area, annoying and relentless yet, not incapacitating. For the next few weeks that followed, I found it was just constant, and not getting better. I continued to see the chiropractor and just about weekly now, I was getting regular massages. I would talk to both practitioners who tried their best, to give me relief, and not really knowing why my shoulder was not responding. I heard things like, "it's probably bursitis, or tendonitis." Some said, "well you know when we get a little older, things just do not always work the way they used too." Believe me, I felt like things were not working the way they used to, but I also expect things to get better, and nothing I was doing was helping.

The first signs of this, started in January that year, and now well into March my right shoulder began to stiffen. Nearly 3 full months, it was still so annoying, and yet it seemed I did not have the same range of motion. No health care provider I had gone to see about my shoulder was much help. Everyone felt like it was a strained muscle or ligament, and if I would just give it a rest and be patient, surely it would get better in time. I tried all types of sports pain relief creams and gels with only temporary success. Almost 4 months into this, my range of motion was becoming obvious, and I could no longer straighten out my arm to the side or over my head. How odd it seemed, from having just a little pain to now much restriction, and the pain was getting worse by the day. In the daytime, as I moved around, the pain was not so bad. I had trouble using my arm much because it was so tight, but at night, the pain was becoming unbearable. I would go to sleep and in the middle of the night, it was as if my arm fell asleep and went from pins and needles to excruciating painful feeling one has as the blood just rolls back into the arm. My shoulder felt like it was on fire. Nothing seemed to help at this point. It made no sense to me how I could go on like this with an arm that just was not working and the pain getting worse, but at night more so than the daytime when I was active. I searched all over the internet to figure out, what causes such a shoulder problem, and what could I do to get relief or fix it.

Also, being a registered nurse, I felt like I should have known what to do and how to treat a little issue like this. I have years working in healthcare, treating many patients through all types of surgical procedures and recoveries, and certainly this was nothing so significant. I began to explore options to bring relief to my debilitating joint on a regular basis. Trips to the chiropractor were several times a week, and now a massage just to the upper body, neck, and affected shoulder two or three times weekly. Both the chiropractor and massage therapist began pointing out that my scapula was looking deformed and different from the other side. They seemed as knowledgeable as I in trying to figure out what was happening to my joint and despite all the work we were doing, the shoulder had a mind of its own and was locking down.

I looked at other types of healing creams, oils, and holistic treatment. My chiropractor used a TENS unit on my upper back, so I looked and found a mini battery-operated one from the local pharmacy that I tried, and it fit perfectly onto my shoulder and scapula area. The one I found was described as a lower back & hip TENS unit, but the pad was perfectly shaped to use all over the shoulder, scapula, deltoid, and bicep. I began using it throughout the day and into the evening, falling asleep with it on, giving just an edge of relief. If I woke up at night, I hit the little button and it would ease the hot burning pain all inside my shoulder. Now the pain had started to run into my bicep and triceps. Again, pain worse in the evening. Waking up in the middle of the night, the shooting pains of my bicep felt like it was on fire. The non-stop pain and irritation of this was just overwhelming to me.

I continued with massages, but found my body was too tight and stiff to carry on with chiropractic care for a little while. Finding acupuncture, was a bit of help to reduce some of the pain, if anything for a few hours during and after the treatment. I just could not get that long of a break, and with such limited movement, I began to call my arm, "my chicken wing." As the shoulder became more and more locked down, the nerves and tendons would stretch beyond their normal range and cause moments of nerve pain shooting down into my fingers.

I scoured the shelves of nutritional and holistic stores. I found Emu oil, and magnesium oil to help give some level of nurturing to my tissues, and joint. None really did the trick, but they seemed to give some relief. Either that, or I was just in so much pain, I mentally felt better after massaging it into my skin.

During this time, I still worked fulltime, because I simply did not think it would go on this long, and I kept telling myself, I just had to work through it. Clearly, I had no "injury," in my mind so how could it be this debilitating for so long? Let me mention the beginning of the mental breakdown of my resilience to this issue. It was hard for me as an independent working mom, to keep myself going as this frozen shoulder was taking a toll on my being. Without realizing it, FS robbed me of energy, and I was feeling exhausted all the time. I just did not relate to how this all started and had taken over my life and my body. Any chance I could, I felt like I needed rest or a nap. I thought it was just because the pain kept me awake or jarred me awake at night. On a day off, I would sleep for 2-3hrs mid-day. I had no idea how to get a hold of this or to turn things around. I felt irritable often, and just could not enjoy anything. My poor family had no idea how to handle the situation, so they were of little help to my issue simply because they felt helpless.

Well into 6 months, I could just hardly take the pain any longer. I had been such a perfect patient to myself. I rested it, I rehabbed it, I nurtured it, I massaged it, I did everything I could for my shoulder, and it only seemed to be getting worse, not better. My routine was just full of hot showers to loosen up, massages, creams, oils, pain relieving gels into and around the joint, and then apply my TENS unit in the AM and moving it around the shoulder and scapula all day to keep the muscle passively moving. I had come home from work, just exhausted from the whole thing, and later, go back out and to the gym for what I called my light rehab workout. Almost daily, I did what I could to keep active either biking, walking and lifting weights, primarily on my unaffected extremities. At this stage, I could hardly lift a one, or two- pound weight on my affected arm. One doctor I went to suggested keeping the other body parts moving, and I would still gain benefits on my affected side, so I took that to heart in hopes of recovering faster. By now, I had complete muscle wasting of both my bicep and triceps, showing no signs of recovery despite all the work I had done to keep it going. This was my dominant side too, so with every attempt to use my arm, I was now met with excruciating pain. I learned quickly what a "zinger" means. It is a jaw dropping shooting pain that feels like when you hit your crazy bone. It comes without warning when you startle the arm in any way. When an occasion presented itself to shake someone's hand, I shuddered as the whole experience was just monumental, and trying to explain my ordeal was just not something I could begin or share over a handshake. I would brace myself for it, to try to minimize the encounter, or find alternatives to just nod or say hi to people, for fear of them seeing how limited I had become, because on the outside I did not want people asking what did I do to myself, as I had absolutely no clue, and was afraid of the Zinger!

LOOKING FOR EXPERT MEDICAL HELP

Six months in and not being able to take it any longer, I tried to get into an orthopedic office to help me figure out what to do. I had given it enough time, and despite my great ideas to heal holistically, nothing was fixing the shoulder. Again, working in the business of healthcare, I reached out to one of our orthopedic surgeons to set up a time for a visit. I had already suffered so long, I called to make an appointment. The receptionist said, "ok, he can see you in 5 weeks." She had to be kidding! I could not possibly stand it any longer. I must be a candidate for an urgent appointment. The pain was intolerable now, and I would have to get in sooner. Did she not know, I must need surgical intervention?! I did not know what had happened to my shoulder, or what was going on, but I had to have someone get in there and fix it, the pain was just killing me. No, even with a network of healthcare providers in my work, I could not get in to see the surgeon any sooner, and I would need to have pictures of my shoulder so get ready to wait.

Let me see what I could do in the meantime. Now, trying to speed the process, I reached out to my chiropractor hoping for his help to order an x-ray or MRI. He gave me the order and a place to go that could get me in right away.

As I was scheduling the MRI, and waiting for the orthopedic visit, I had to take a trip out of town on a long flight. During the trip, I came across an article in the airline magazine that talked about stem cell treatments for joint dysfunction and healing. The minute I landed I made a call. I had no idea if this could help, but I could just not take the 24/7 pain of it any longer, and still did not know what was causing it. I called about the treatment and they seemed very knowledgeable with all types of joint issues, and said I could come in for a consultation, and if the doctor felt he could treat my issue, we could plan same day care for it. I was ready. It was to the point, I wanted to cut my arm off, it was so bad. The office was so understanding, she had me set up to visit just over a week later, and to make sure I could get evaluated she recommended coming with the MRI and report.

EMOTIONAL & MENTAL HEALTH FIRST 6 MONTHS

Up through this point of wrangling this condition on my own, I have yet to mention the deterioration of my psyche as no one around me saw an issue. I looked normal, healthy, active just quieter perhaps and a bit removed. I was mentally and physically exhausted because whatever this issue was in my shoulder just took every ounce of energy to keep myself going. Who would get that? What did I do? No clue. What exactly happened or changed that one joint in my body malfunctioned and basically shut down? If I were to describe a depressed feeling or overwhelming sense of helplessness would be an understatement. This issue had taken over my whole being. At the time, I did not know all the inner workings of my shoulder and how it could lead to exhaustion. I just knew I was living inside a personal hell and those around me had no clue. Tired all the time I just about fell out daily. I began to look at myself and emotionally could not fight the fight however small. I had moments I would cry for no reason. So I thought, I think I was scared thinking how could I feel so bad, what had I done, what had I not done, and how did this all happen and I was not even there for the "reason or event," that must have done this to me. I began thinking, was it a tumor in my shoulder, could I have cancer, was this fixable, treatable, much less even curable and fast!

Those closest to me did not understand, could not understand, even what was there to understand? I was a mess. It is one thing the known. You break an arm, and get it fixed. It takes time. In general, it will heal 6-10 weeks and you know, up to this moment, I felt I either missed my window to "fix" it, or I must have something uncurable. The time seemed to just drag on forever with this issue and I just could find one single answer that made a bit of sense. I knew then I had to be not just physically beaten, but my emotional state felt like it too, would never recover. I did not have a big support system, but my one major support was my husband. He never doubted it was more than just something was not right, he encouraged me to seek answers and treatment to figure it out. He made my emotional state better by simply not judging me. He helped wherever he could and most nights or when we were together provided that emotional component to just let me scream, cry, or complain how unfair was this situation, and most important he helped me to rest or be there to just keep me from being alone with my mind in this complex physical situation that wrecked emotional havoc nearly as bad as the physical pain.

ALTERNATIVE TREATMENT

The day was here, and I flew into town to check out this treatment with anxious anticipation. The pain in my shoulder was off the scale, and I figured there could not be anything to top it or make it worse. I was ready to cut my arm off or something if I had not found some way to relieve the pain in some fashion. I felt like nothing to lose and since I had not found anyone to treat this issue so far, I was at least looking and willing to try something beyond massage, and creams, and medication. I had asked my son to take me to this visit, because I planned to get something done to this shoulder no matter what it was going to be. I arrived at the office, and I waited with several others who were in different phases of stem cell treatment. Casually talking with others waiting, they seemed to speak of the positive results they were having to other parts of their body with painful issues. One had a knee treatment, and the other just beginning treatment for a lower back issue. I went in for my consult, and armed with my MRI results, the doctor began looking at the pictures and tried moving my right arm. He had brought in his assistant and discussing my extremely limited range of motion. Not surprised at all by my limitations and review of the MRI, he said, "You have a frozen shoulder. One of the worst I have seen in a long time..."

"What is a frozen shoulder?" I asked. I told him, I have been a nurse for an exceptionally long time and never heard of such a thing. He said, "well, the technical term is adhesive capsulitis." He reviewed my MRI and said there is all kinds of things going on in your shoulder. There were to small tears to the labrum. A full thickness tear, about 20% through it, known as a rotator tear. Bursitis- type of irritation as well, and all of that creates a perfect medium for the ball and socket joint of the shoulder to lock down. So now I wondered, what will stem cells do? How could this possibly help. In my world, a rotator tear I knew was usually surgically repaired, with weeks of rehabilitation and immobilization. Now I thought of one of my cross-fit instructors who had been out for weeks with surgery and a shoulder immobilizer. I came all this way and would still have to wait weeks for the orthopedic surgeon. I started to wonder if this initial onset of FS came as a result of an undetected rotator tear from one of my earlier cross-fit classes. I could not say for sure, but it is a theory. Now, this doctor, explained how stem cells would do the job, and I would not need surgery. He had trained for years in sports and orthopedic medicine in the Ukraine, and began doing research, and found how stem cells create healing at the cellular level. When injected into areas of pain, inflammation, and issues, the stem cells go to work decreasing the inflammation, and promote healing without the need to go in and cut away or repair rotator tears inside the body with sutures or clips.

He described the way to retrieve the cells and how it is done using one's own blood or adipose tissue. It would take just a little while to get it set up, but it could all be done same day. No need for a long preparation or need to come back to the office, but to be effective, I did need to have a series of at least 3-4 treatments 2 days apart. My response was a resounding, "Yes! Let us get started!" I had 2 other problems. Time and money. I needed to fly back so I could get back to work, and stem cells were new to marketplace and not paid up front by insurance. I only had enough for 2 treatments and could not stay long enough in town either. The physician was very understanding and suggested to try the two, to see if I have an improvement. I could always add more later, and I might get lucky to have some benefit or full recovery. It was worth a try.

STEM CELL TREATMENT

He had me go into the treatment area where they drew blood and removed just a syringe full of adipose tissue. It took just under 30 minutes to get things together and then I waited till my own cells were spun down and ready to be injected. Just about 40 minutes later, they were set, and I returned into the treatment room for an injection into my painful shoulder. It was not the most pleasant feeling to have an injection into the joint, but my day to day pain was well off the chart over 10, so knowing this could end that and take the pain away made it tolerable. First, he numbed the area with local anesthetic, then gave it some time to take effect. The staff really helped me get through the preparation. They were very understanding, knowing the pain so many people are going through, this is just the icing on the cake. When injecting into a joint, there is a lot of feeling of pressure, because the fluid fills the area and the goal is to get enough in there to loosen things up and get to healing. While he was in there injecting, he said he felt the tightness of adhesions of tissue all around inside the joint. The fluid really got in there and filled the capsule. I was in a bit of discomfort, but not so bad knowing this could really work and get my shoulder back on the right track to healing. After he finished the injection, the therapist with him, put several ice packs all around the shoulder and had me rest for about 20 minutes to help with discomfort and swelling. After the treatment was done, I waited and received instructions to return in 2 days for a second series of treatment, going through exactly what he had just done, and said this would be most beneficial to resolve my frozen shoulder. I returned 2 days later and went through the exact same process. I do not know if it is because I knew what to expect, or if my shoulder was starting to have greater feeling from the treatment, but this time it was even a bit more uncomfortable. Still, I believed this was such an amazing alternative to any type of surgical intervention. Relieved it was all over, the doctor and physical therapist went over my course of treatment for when I got home. In a day or two, they told me to begin moving it, stretching and doing all the things I normally do. I told them, that is not much because for the last 7 or 8 months, I just could not do much with it progressively freezing and causing so much pain. He said, that is how frozen shoulder works. It goes through 3 stages, and from the point of freezing, to now frozen, this will accelerate the "thaw." I asked if a physical therapy plan was needed, and he said no, just keep it moving as much as you can, and if you do, it will all resolve. At that moment, my shoulder was painful, and I could not imagine how it would resolve on its own. I went home that day and just thought about what he said and hoped it would work. With the first and second treatment done, I wondered if it was going to really make a difference. The second injection left me in a bit more pain and I just had hoped I had not wasted a few thousand dollars that gave me no guarantees now. Feeling rough all over, I went back to settle in and rest before I left to fly home the next morning. I did prop myself up and iced the shoulder. I really gave it time to let all those cells in there a chance to settle in and go to work. For the next 24 hours I just rested and moved around a little as instructed to just let things gel inside that joint.

GETTING RESULTS

I waited a day or so and started doing just what the doctor said to do. Moving my arm and trying to "test it" was my plan to see if I had any hope to get it back to normal. I continued over the next few days and realized if nothing else, the pain in my shoulder, especially at night had almost gone away completely. I had slept through the night the last two nights. I no longer woke up in the middle of the night with excruciating pain, like a hot knife in my shoulder and down my bicep and triceps. The doctor had told me, the pain becomes so bad, as it is "freezing," because the joint overstretches, and much of the soft tissue with it, the ligaments and tendons become stretched beyond where they belong. Some of them develop micro tears and with everything so inflamed, the nerves all around the area become affected too. At night, when the body is at rest, and blood pressure is at its lowest, all the nerve endings flair and the tissue just is on "fire." That makes sense now, because during the day, activity is less painful and moving around made it feel a bit more normal, except movement became so restricted and finally, "frozen."

Now with pain diminished and feeling like I was healing, I began to test it pushing my limits with better responsiveness in the shoulder joint. I was not doing anything crazy, except moving and stretching to the point I felt comfortable. I continued to become more active again and started back to the chiropractor who was pleased with my progress. He said, whatever I did was working, and to continue to move and gently exercise as movement on one side will certainly help my affected side. I also found massage immensely helpful to really get motion back into the shoulder. Visiting the massage therapist twice a week for focused effort on the upper body, shoulder and neck, was getting it to start to make some crackly movement and motion. She would work deep into and around the shoulder and armpit. There are numerous trigger points along the under arm and side chest wall. The pain was nearly resolved, just a bit of soreness, which reminded me not to overdo things, but gave me a chance to rest at night and see progress daily. She also added some stretches with the massage after releasing each pressure point.

My fitness routine continued with running on the treadmill or cycle class. I usually attended 30-45-minute intervals and then used a variety of weight equipment focusing on my unaffected side. I also used a giant exercise ball to do abdominal work and stretches. Gradually, I reintroduced weights on the affected arm starting with 1-2 pounds, and moving to 5 pounds, then 8 pounds over the next few weeks after I thawed and progressed from there.

I was just hitting nine months of limited mobility as things finally began to clear in my right shoulder. What the doctor said, I found true, and I did not do anything rigorous or painful or dramatic to get my shoulder moving. Instead, I treated it gingerly, and kept it moving as much as possible. Finally, I had so much crackling and clearing that I could feel my shoulder breaking up on the inside and gained my range of motion back to the joint. It really was amazing, and to have gone through something so crazy like this and not knowing what to expect from the pain off the charts and locking down of the joint, to finally moving again, left me crying tears of joy.

RECOVERY FAST FORWARD

There is nothing quite so unnerving and debilitating as what they call it, "frozen shoulder" aka adhesive capsulitis. Getting to this point along with the pain and affliction, I also found myself become a frozen shoulder, FS for short, guru! The literature at the time was limited. Now there is more to find on the internet for this crazy condition. During my time with my first frozen shoulder, I searched to find answers and found I was discovering and sharing with others in similar situations all over the world. In the 9 months of weathering this process, I found social media to be a source of support. There are Facebook groups I joined for those who find themselves with this unknown shoulder ailment. The groups are well over 2000 to nearly 4000 sufferers strong all over the world it seems. They share stories, ask questions, look for answers, and support each other as each finds their way to hope, and healing. What I learned and tips and ideas are what I hope to share here so that others who find themselves with FS, adhesive capsulitis can learn and know they are not alone and there is light at the end of the tunnel for this situation. I seemed to develop this as a 50th birthday present, with no real origin or injury. I seemed to have some basic characteristics. I was in a general age range where this occurs, female, perimenopausal, and undergoing an extreme amount of personal stress. It seems those who are also diabetic, or with any type of autoimmune issue has an increased risk. Those who have a diet that includes sugar, processed foods, or otherwise not super healthy can also increase their odds to develop this condition. Others who have had an injury or shoulder, neck or breast and lymphatic surgery also increase the likelihood of developing adhesive capsulitis or freezing too, related to limited mobility that will irritate the shoulder joint and surrounding tissues. The most troubling aspect of this condition, syndrome, illness, or whatever you might liken it to is there is still no verdict out on a specific cause. Triggers are what I have found to be what starts the inflammatory process going. A trigger being an insult to the body. Sometimes directly to the shoulder itself like trauma, surgery, or an injection in that joint area. Other more general triggers could be a long-standing illness or virus that wears down the immune system or initiates a response from the immune system that puts it into overdrive setting off the shoulder joint. There are other disease processes that have been noted like diabetic, lupus, or other issues that have an auto-immune component that again, seem to trigger an overdrive response landing in one or both shoulders. As in my case, I never dreamed I be one of the few to have it hit my other shoulder. The data at the time indicates less than 20% who are affected with frozen shoulder will end up with it in the other shoulder. I thought I had great odds. There are several who end up in a dreadful case of bilateral frozen shoulder meaning they develop it in both shoulders at the same time, or the second one hits before the first one is resolved. Currently, there is not enough research or data out there to confirm or deny once you have frozen shoulder you may or may not get it again. I am really hoping that those of us who have encountered this beast once, much less twice in the case of it hitting both shoulders never are affected again. To that point I will mention a bit later, it is worth considering how the frozen shoulder resolves. If in fact it is possible, could it be a shoulder that goes through its course, and does not dramatically try to break the cycle through surgery or joint manipulation have a better chance of permanent remission rather than a recurrence years later? We will have to see the research over time. Throughout this journey and you will see with my second shoulder, the emotional component is key. When afflicted with such an event, and not knowing what one is dealing with is traumatic enough; however, the steadying of physical and emotional aspects with no end in sight or a promise or hope for recovery can be maddening. I suggest having witnessed the psyche unravel, a consideration for support measures to one who finds themselves with this affliction. It could be a support group, private or using social media, a counselor, or a close family member or friend whom you might familiarize them with all you are learning and share the research and this information with them so they can know how important their non-judgmental approach and support is needed to get you through this very long journey. I cannot say with certainty each individual case because again, just like the triggers, the recoveries vary based on the successes and responses of the immune system and joint function.

FAST FORWARD (FS2) THE "OTHER" SHOULDER IS AFFECTED

3 years nearly to the day, my left shoulder began with an unusually odd tightness around the scapula on a cold, rainy January morning. I could not believe for a minute after the months, nearly a year of healing that without an injury or a cause, my non-dominant side was getting that "feeling" like the other side. This time, not even the possibility of a workout injury or a stretch or tear from an unusual position, it just began. Yet, we always look for clues and causes, and I must say I did have a lot of stress on my plate from a career and family standpoint. Stress alone, can cause physical symptoms in many of us, so I gave that the reason for striking my second side and knowing having had the right side affected, if the theory was true, it was the up and coming left side's turn to develop this nasty affliction. Armed with the toolkit of remedies, I began my second frozen shoulder (FS) journey. So, in the rest of this book,

I will give you some of my language and terms for how I worked through not one, but two frozen shoulders successfully, without heavy medications, blind shoulder manipulation under anesthesia, or surgery. I can tell you frozen shoulder is extremely physically painful and inordinately debilitating. The emotional and mental component of stress placed enduring this illness is often why I encourage others to take time for themselves to nurture and heal their bodies both physically and emotionally. The other aspects to consider are these:

1. How did it develop, without warning, slow and insidious, or was it a result of a traumatic event, fall, or post-surgical intervention of shoulder or upper body area as in the case of breast surgery, or lymphatic surgery?

2. What type of treatment model are you seeking to find healing?

HOLISTIC VS PAIN MGMT. OR SURGICAL INTERVENTIONS

The way FS develops may be reason why one may choose a more aggressive approach over another. If it comes on much like one develops the flu, or tennis elbow, just a non-specific journey of immobility, it usually means that is how it will run the course and most often can run 9 months to 18 months just keeping comfortable, nurturing, and being active towards resolution. Depending on how quickly a plan of attack is started, there are some people who have suffered even longer. If it is an abrupt onset, from a trauma, fall, or post-surgery, greater intervention quicker might be needed to help undo some mechanical trauma or damage from the event. It is how you decide to manage the course of treatment and finding the practitioners you want to work with to get you to your goal. Until the pain sparks lack of sleep and constant throbbing with total inability to function, many will not understand why you need to learn about FS before your in the throes of such maddening anguish. Had I not been met with delays for more aggressive treatment, I may not have chosen or stuck with the holistic approach. Also, knowing there was some rotator tear involvement, I also was of the understanding all tears required surgery. That is not always the case. In this journey, I discovered and focused on how to best heal the joint without further complication of surgical intervention or medication side effects. This may not be what you end up doing, and you may even mix several combinations that work for you. Just be sure you are well informed. Beyond the physical component, the emotional component must be considered. Can you endure the course and work through balancing nurture, and tenacity to manage through the pain in order to get to the other side of healing? If you have ever experienced childbirth, until the first one is imminent one may think it can be managed naturally without medication or even surgical intervention. However, nature does not always allow for our best intentions and medications and surgery have a place and can be lifesaving. These recommendations, and my approach are not a test of wills, only a way to inspire and insure if you can pursue this method, you can make it and fully recover. If you find barriers and obstacles that cannot be overcome, do not give up and use whatever available through a trusted practitioner or program that will get you results. No matter the course, frozen shoulder can resolve and can be treated. How you set your mind to work it through is one aspect not to overlook or discount in the process. Much like labor, we are not all cut out for a natural experience. To do so is not a failure, just a different approach. My background and career have afforded the opportunity to know how to test, try, and move that has prepared me to get through this twice with some additional medical intervention, and now I have been able to coach and support others. Most important of all, if you are getting results, keep going. If you are not, continue to explore and seek information and guidance along the way. There are many who can help from a variety of modalities. My goal is to let you know that this, is real, and you can and will heal.

FREEZING, FROZEN, THAW PHASES

Generally said, the onset of adhesive capsulitis (frozen shoulder) starts with the shoulder not feeling normal. It may be a twinge, a feeing of thickness, a slight irritation or little pain along the scapula. It is not a noticeable problem in the beginning. If it begins after a fall, or accident, or surgery, similarly it may not be discovered as the general swelling from these conditions and limited movement is expected. With injury or surgery, often the plan is to keep the area isolated and some of this lack of movement from the initial plan is what triggers the FS response to begin lock down. Early mobility is a double-edged sword in this case, so for those already dealing with trauma or postop recovery, the holistic approach will have its challenges because this type of FS seems to stem from the very inflammatory response to the tissues injured or repaired surgically or around the joint area itself. Some of the information and techniques in here described along with an idiopathic FS, can augment care but chances are the duration and treatment will probably best benefit from a more traditional orthopedic approach and a practitioner or MT or PT who can keep moving the arm passively until the strength is regained to do so independently. Tip: recovery may create soreness or post treatment pain, but during a therapy session, motion should always be stopped up to the point of pain and not greater. Too often, the term, "no pain no gain," is not meant for healing of an injury. This seems to be what I have found with some interventionists I tried and fired. The eager, aggressive approach should not bring the person to tears or be so sore during or following any treatment, they cringe to want to come back. If that is the case, have enough wherewithal to evaluate yourself. Are you anxious and afraid not giving treatment a chance or are you working to the best you can and feel pushed to beyond the point of pain? There is nothing wrong with re-evaluating progress and going in a new direction or with someone new. It may save you time, money, and you might progress faster.

As the days and weeks press on in the freezing phase, the same daily tasks become more difficult. The shoulder does not move easily and often limits of overhead movement or external rotation of the arm begins to shorten. In the throes of full adhesive capsulitis, FS there is no point to pushing to keep range of motion improving or aggressive therapy. The phases and stages of this syndrome or illness if you will, really cannot be stopped or halted regardless of claims to immediately release the shoulder. It is a 3 phased systemic event that gets to this point and once locked down, know it can be weeks to months to begin to thaw into the next phase of unfreezing. It is in freezing that often, based on the time someone's shoulder has been affected that surgical interventions may be discussed.

For the benefit of mentioning a few there are two procedures typically done with a frozen shoulder. The first is manipulation under anesthesia. The second is known as a shoulder arthroscopy. With arthroscopy, they can view into the joint through a lens. The joint may be viewed, scraped and cleaned up removing scar tissue, and doing any type of repair that may be needed to the tissue. Some know it as "keyhole surgery." The manipulation under anesthesia is still a surgical approach, but it is where there are no incisions. With surgery, there are many considerations, and if the time is right for you, an aggressive approach like this could be what you might prefer. With the manipulation, MUA, a person is heavily sedated not usually completely anesthetized. The arm is moved around in a variety of positions diligently to blindly break up adhesions and scar tissue to release the "freeze" of the joint. Often, with both surgical interventions, a block is placed, so for about 8-12 hours the area is numb to pain. Each of the procedures can provide results. Just be sure you ask good questions about the specifics of what each procedure entails, downtime, long and short complications, and outcomes of those complications. Neither should be entered into lightly. One of the reasons I chose to not go the surgical route is I had seen too many experiences in my surgical career where some of those complications came to light. It does not mean they are not an alternative, especially for frozen shoulders that have gone well beyond a year. It does mean that when you consider the course of freezing, frozen, and thaw, one might be just around the corner from the next progression and either of the surgical interventions will create a significant inflammatory response. This response often normal will delay current progress and often feel like a step back the first initial week or two. In other cases, either mobility is not going forward and a refreeze develops or the inflammatory response is overzealous and delays healing also. Other complications can be significant and best discussed with your provider. It is a very personal and individualized choice not to be taken lightly. With the intense and almost traumatizing pain, decisions at this phase are challenging. I would recommend giving it a few days to decide from the discussion with your provider, and to get a second or third opinion. The one thing that I have learned and continue to see is, once a person is already at this freezing point, an intervention like this does have potential to create a "re-freeze." The refreeze is not because the procedure did or did not go as planned, it is just the body's immune response is doing what it is supposed to do and create an inflammatory response to an "insult" to the system. In this case, it means it is not a new frozen shoulder or even a complication, it is just going to take a bit longer or an extended time to recover to thaw. What you need to consider is how long you have been suffering and how long are you willing to keep going if you have not had improvements to thaw yet and you might be well over a year. Then another 4-12 weeks to get there with this type of intervention is just like I said, staying the course and persevering it through to the end. If you are having progress, slow, but progress it may be worth continuing to up your tenacity and see it through before shifting to surgery then. You need to weigh all options.

That said, the other techniques for help with frozen shoulder can be injections of cortisone, hydrodilitation, stem cells or platelet rich plasma. I will mention them all here, but would be remiss, if I did not share my professional thoughts on why I might not recommend them all. Injections remember are not always done the same by any one provider so I cannot say an injection is a failure as the person may not have been the best to inject it. It means go to someone with a great track record and recommendations. The first, cortisone, is a steroidal anti-inflammatory. This is meant to decrease inflammation in the tissue. It is temporary, and again my opinion 50/50 chance to at least minimize the pain. Many have commented of the lasting zinger pain as it sometimes creates nerve irritation which just makes one want to hit the ceiling for hours on end. Some do not experience that at all. The other, of more concern, is that of the lasting effects on the actual tissues injected. It has the mechanics to be harmful to the tissues and with each subsequent injection, it may stop the inflammatory process from working or moving forward. In this case there is no option to continue injections and it is noted in most literature also that no more than 3 injections into the joint are recommended over time. For those that are diabetic, it has shown to wreck -havoc with blood sugar levels, sometimes temporarily or causing a shift to elevate requiring follow up medical care. Of note, it also is in some literature, and physician experience, once the inflammatory process is halted, surgery becomes nearly the most only helpful option because there is no inflammation process left to help heal. It is my experience of my career only, that I share why I would prefer other options, if not just letting time take its course as opposed to diving prematurely into surgery.

Hydrodilitation is a way to take a saline type injection into the joint to flush, irrigate, and hydrate to relieve the stickiness of the adhesions in hopes to rebalance and open the shoulder joint capsule. This treatment has been noted to work in many cases, but without the literature, and enough subjects to test validity again is only offered as a means to explain and share options that currently exist out there and only in some parts of the world. The final injection duo is known as PRP, platelet rich plasma and stem cell injections. Since having had these myself I of course will share how and why I found them to work well. There still is limited research so this is where you need to investigate and research to decide for yourself. The PRP is used by withdrawing blood from your vein and then spinning it down so the platelets full of stem cells can be used to inject into the joint directly. Usually the joint is numbed locally, and then the joint is filled about 10cc full of the PRP. In many of the joint injections the feeling is "full or pressure." The goal behind the PRP is to have the powerful cells go to work regenerating health cells to rebuild the tissue and use strong anti-inflammatory properties to reduce the swelling and breakdown the adhesions. Similarly, the stem cells pulled from adipose tissue in the abdomen or bone marrow are even stronger and the potency is where the ability exists to create dramatic healing. The abdominal adipose is not a big deal to remove. Local injection to the site, and a large needle withdraws the fat cells in a 30-60cc syringe looks much like chicken fat found on a chicken breast at the store. In the research you will find many regenerative programs popping up across the country. Not all use your own spun down cells. The later I have not seen as consistent effect as alternative cells are used. Typically, these can come from other live hosts often embryonic cord blood. The reason they have a lesser benefit to work 100% is because the body may find them to be foreign and reject the powerful help intended to give and be inert in the effort. Back to the research though as, this is advancing daily and what may not work today is still being tested and improved so the more learned and studied could show future promise.

An area to explore is a procedure typically done in Canada and only a few streams popping up internationally is called the "OATS" procedure. It too is also a specific manipulation technique from a practice expert in Canada. It is believed it is done by a Doctor of Osteopathic or Chiropractor trained. This being so remote to myself in the USA, and equally less researched and almost unbelievable, I did not explore this too much. A one stop pop and go of the joint and without any type of analgesia or anesthesia was just not something I felt logical or worth considering. I am of the mindset though many may have felt similarly to my approach as it really deviates from the typical medical Western model. I would be remiss not to suggest exploring all options, and if it is possible maybe this procedure once greater studied and or a larger group of participants and seeing successes could be a viable option. So, I say explore them all to find solutions to keep you sane, while moving toward health restoring your shoulder.

TOOLKIT OF IDEAS FOR NURTURING

TENS Unit (transcutaneous electrical nerve stimulation) – this can be extremely beneficial for a variety of reasons with the shoulder. The TENS unit be applied all over the muscle areas of the shoulder, scapula, and latissimus dorsi to ease the intensity of frozen shoulder pain. Some do not find pain relief much with the TENS unit, but there is an added healing benefit which provides increased blood flow to the area. This increased blood flow assists with healing and the inflammatory process. It is a great way to "passively" work the muscles. This work allows rest of the body, yet the muscles are still working to keep the area healthy. As I noted earlier, I was able to find a "mini" tens unit that is battery operated and can be worn throughout the day and night. In doing so, one is not tied to a machine and it is similar to having a passive physical therapy session anytime of day which is extremely helpful because with frozen shoulder, unlike an injury or surgical insult, rest is the key. Frozen shoulder heals better and progressively well when there is frequent movement. This is also the main benefit to helping the shoulder at night or sleeping, as at rest, the pain flairs. Use of a TENS, needs some guidance because it is not to just place it on the shoulder and go. The areas need to rotate off and on and at intervals. Looking around in many over the counter stores where pain relivers are sold, one can find a few different brands of the battery-operated units for hips, knees, back, and recently the shoulder. At the back of the book, specific questions related to this or other holistic options can be emailed to me for further follow up or where to find things.

Heat and Cold packs- temperature relief is personal decision to find what works. Normally ice is used in acute injuries and a few days later heat applied for healing. With frozen shoulder, it is not so specific. Inflammation does well and responds to ice often. Heat is soothing and increased blood flow to the area and can equally create a healing response. In the case and the course of frozen shoulder many find relief alternating the two. Remembering to check skin, sensation, and always remember to keep on usually no greater than 20-minute intervals.

With heat, the use of showers, warm pools, steam and dry saunas can provide relief and should be utilized during the freezing, frozen, and thaw journey. Just as a note, the steam room and hot tub were places that allowed a deep penetrating heat to get into the joint and facilitate a real support to thaw when used frequently.

Topical pain relievers, creams, gels, sprays – There are a ton of creams, gels, salves, sprays that can be tried to find one that helps. Of a particular note, are the heated and cooling ones that give a therapeutic feel to touch those nerves/pain receptors. There are intense ones creating such a heat response like Cepacian that are great to try, just use delicately and carefully do not do activities that create sweat or go out in the sun. If used in a quiet, dry environment that super deep heat can feel miraculous even for just a few hours. Magnesium oil or spray is great for muscle repair and soothing to the shoulder or injured area. Emu oil with its healing and restorative properties is another solution to try when looking for topical support to the entire shoulder area neck or back.

Many other balms and creams can provide similar benefit and should be explored. One of the reasons these are recommended and preferred over ingested pain medication is to not add injury to the gut and other complications that will come only to aggravate the already devastating condition of frozen shoulder that lead to complications like constipation, fatigue, diarrhea, headache, abdominal pain, depression, blood sugar spikes, and others.

Over the Counter Pain Relievers and Prescription Medications-this is an area of personal exploration. As being a nurse and holistic advanced practitioner, I chose a course of alternatives avoiding most ingestible medication. Short-term mild pain relievers can certainly help. The only reason I caution the what, why, and length is simply because of my concern with other conditions that can be exacerbated, and even created by longer term use of counter and prescribed meds for pain, inflammation, nerve pain and others. Recommendations are to find what you can live with and what you cannot. If you find the need to have medicinal support, do so with a goal to find alternatives to manage perhaps heat, shower or massage as well. Medications, especially pain medication, minimally touches the pain as frozen shoulder pushes to freezing. Nerve pain can be debilitating and often with movement and use of a TENS, heat or ice a better result can be achieved than using a pain medication NSAIDS or narcotic. Again, this is individual, but most often say the medication just does not take the pain away enough to sleep or think at points of the freezing process. For this reason, it is so important to find multiple modalities.

Pillows, support pads, snugglies- in the most debilitating moments of frozen shoulder finding and using any type of pillow device to prop the arms to sleep upright or to position in and around body to maneuver a side lying position are critical to your toolkit.

Natural Supplement Corner- See the list below, and by far it is not all inclusive. Many of the items below are what were found helpful to heal the gut, or to support the inflammation process and decrease the body's inflammation. This can take a whole section on nutrition to heal naturally and will only just touch on key ingredients.

Ashwagandha- helpful with normalizing imbalances and stressors in the body. Decreases inflammation and stimulates immune activity.

Curcumin- member of the ginger family and contains turmeric. Powerful anti-inflammatory and strong antioxidant.

Turmeric – a spice that eases joint pain, inflammation, and stiffness. It has curcumin in it.

Green tea- full of antioxidants that help with blood flow, decrease inflammation, and improve vessel function to support cells.

White Willow Bark- helpful for relieving pain like arthritis, back pain, and joint pain.

Pycnogenol (Maritime Pine Bark)- helpful to help with muscle pain and supports antioxidant properties of immune support.

Capsaicin (Chili pepper)- strong topical analgesic and helps with nerve or neuralgia pain.

Boswellia – powerful anti-inflammatory and painkiller

Black Pepper- high in antioxidants, anti-inflammatories, and supports decreased joint inflammation.

Cat's Claw (Uncaria Tomentosa)- useful to fight infections and fight infection

Rosemary- strong antioxidant and anti-inflammatory also supports neurological function

Cloves- strong antioxidant properties and fights bacteria.

Ginger- known for stimulating circulation and a strong anti-inflammatory. It has been used in arthritic conditions to inhibit cytokines or messengers in the chemical immune system. It also benefits stomach upsets and soothes digestion and gastric irritation.

Cinnamon- a powerful antioxidant and super food ingredient, it can be powerful to fight infection and repair tissue damage.

Peppermint- (oil) antiviral and antifungal uses and analgesia-ingested. Topically, can also be used as a pain-reliever.

Apple Cider Vinegar- helpful with lowering blood sugar and digestion demand. Useful support in improving cleaning the gut and improving digestive function.

Diets to Alkalize Body- why alkaline diet changes are potentially beneficial because a diet that is more alkaline has shown in some instances to support internal healing and reduction of inflammation which can lead to disease or chronic issue. There are many books and internet articles to gain insight on how to improve overall well-being by implementing this type of diet to support improvement to those suffering with a frozen shoulder.

Avoid Acidifying body (meats, eggs, cheese, processed foods, breads, pastas)

Decreasing Yeast (candida) Fermented foods such as **sauerkraut, kimchi, kombucha, and keifer** provide the healthy bacteria needed in the gut–the bacteria that will ultimately crowd out Candida.

Foods that kill fungi include **onions, leeks, green apples, ginger, pomegranates, and citrus fruits**.

Essential Oils. **Clove oil, oregano oil and myrrh oil** are all known to be powerful antifungals that can help kill a variety of parasites and fungi in the body, including candida. **Lavender oil** is also known to stop the continued growth of candida and prevent the spread of infection throughout the body

https://www.healthline.com/nutrition/candida-symptoms-treatment#section4

The above website gives a nice summary of how candida can really impact the body's immune system to impair healing and support a lag to healing frozen shoulder. Candida is not our friend.

Detoxifying Body:

https://healthwholeness.com/detox/how-to-detox-your-body/

Detox is really an important aspect to consider in facilitating to rid your body of things that can impair healing. The A's have it. As the above site shares, artichokes, asparagus, and avocados can dramatically improve liver cleanse and function, healthy bile production, and immune boosting.

Apples- Avocados – Beets- Blueberries- Celery-
Cranberries -Cabbage- Flaxseeds- Flaxseed oils -Garlic –
Grapefruit- Kale -Legumes- Lemons- Seaweed- Watercress

These are all great sources of nutrition and clean eating that
can be extremely beneficial to the body's healing, digestion, and
cleansing. When incorporated into a holistic diet routine, much of
what is used to fuel the internal functioning of one's body will have
tremendous effects in fighting and healing systemic and functional
issues.

NEWER TECHNIQUE TO SUPPORT HEALING

Cryotherapy: deep ice/freezing technology to work much like ice packs taking part of the body or entire body to treat with a deep freeze to reduce inflammation. I have personally tried after my frozen shoulders with a muscle tear and found it beneficial. Thoughts to its use with the process of frozen shoulder is certainly something to explore.

https://www.cryotherapytreatments.com/

Lasers for Pain Relief and Healing:

Much research has been done on the deep healing benefits using laser light. This is another treatment I used not for my shoulder but after a significant muscle tear in my hamstring post frozen shoulder days. I think had it been available while I was in the living nightmare of frozen shoulder, the benefits and recovery to heal a torn muscle would have also produced positive benefits. There are many great providers out there offering these treatments and again, to find solutions it is worth exploring. https://www.spineuniverse. com/treatments/physical-therapy/pain-relief-healing-laser-therapy

Photo biomodulation light therapy (red light) Is where cellular stimulation creates ATP activity and stimulates cellular motion and aids in healing. It can be extremely beneficial in tissue healing and decreasing inflammation by the energy created in stimulating circulation. This communication happens by transmission of signals throughout the entire body. Additionally, nitric oxide helps to dilate the blood vessels and improve blood circulation.

https://vielight.com/photobiomodulation/

Dry Saunas: these have several benefits to consider. They boost immune system after being in one for about 15 minutes or so. They increase white blood cell production to fight inflammation and infection. Saunas will stimulate blood flow and improves circulation. These effects all can benefit frozen shoulder if done once a week.

https://www.medicalnewstoday.com/articles/313109# health-myths

Steam Rooms: Many benefits specific to frozen shoulder include improved ability to drive range of motion. The moist heat can really get in and make it easier to stretch and move the body and joints while inside the steam room. It can help with circulation, blood flow and immune responses too. Sweating and cleansing the body is also another way to help to assist in detoxifying too. As with both dry and steam heat, to keep rehydrated as they both pull fluid off and can result in dizzy, light-headed, and headaches if not replenished before, during, and after a session.

https://activatedyou.com/steam-room-benefits/

SURVIVING AND THRIVING BEYOND FROZEN SHOULDER

In looking back at surviving through each frozen shoulder, it was just as much of a mental mission as well as a physical condition to overcome. The wrath of this condition for anyone can be daunting to say the least. It can bring one's own sanity into question in terms of surviving the undulating pain, and longevity of this illness. Understanding it is not typically an injury that needs rehabilitation, but more of a mechanism of an illness to the joint capsule. Considering this, it is important when planning the course of treatment to heal. While much is still not known in terms of the perfect pathway to recovery, it is a journey, and everyone is different. Some can take on this journey, with similar ideas as I, and stay the course nurturing and working with and around the shoulder pain and inflammation to restore the range of motion. Others may find the pain and journey too crippling and look to pain medications, and surgery. While there is not right or best answer knowing what options and what has been tried and successful can be extremely helpful to knowing you are not alone in this journey. When first discovering something was wrong, I was scared and in denial that this had to be fixed and no way could I endure months or longer to heal. It is astounding how this illness grips people and takes them to places mentally that can be so hard, painful, and detrimental to their psyche, and others close to them. It is because it is so silent, that when one is affected first, they do not even understand what is going on as it invades their shoulder and the inflammatory process of their body. Second, it does not look from the outside that anything is wrong with the individual. In the sense as the frozen shoulder develops makes it unbearable to return a handshake or move through the day not knowing the pain coming when a bump to the arm or a zinger ensues. It is such a silent, painful road that it is important to educate and provide insight and resources to those suffering and to those close to them so they can know and understand this intensely painful experience that takes months to years to heal. The most important think to stress is to explore options. Know that there is currently not any one perfect way to diagnose and fix a frozen shoulder. There are several ways to zero in and define and identify one may have an adhesive capsulitis related to no known reason, or it could have manifested from an injury or as a result of a surgery as a secondary event. Some could have it develop as a precursor of an autoimmune issue or underlying disease like diabetes. No matter what, know you are not alone, and looking for solutions, modifying life or staging the marathon to keep a balance of activity and nurturing are entirely a personal choice of going the journey and in the end beating frozen shoulder. My hope for you in reading my journey is to know you can and will see this to the other side of healing and restoring function. My best to you and those around you. Look to the resources included and consider ways to find local providers and solutions in your area.

While I am available as a resource and licensed clinician, know that there are many professionals becoming more educated to treat and guide individuals encountering this mystifying illness to the joint. Be Well and Stay Strong, you will recover....

ABOUT THE AUTHOR

Patti is an advanced practice nurse with a career in nursing well over 30+ years. Much of her time in the surgical arena helped her to learn and understand pathophysiology, working with many well-trained orthopedic surgeons in many hospitals across the USA. She grew in leadership roles and eventually opened a wellness center that catered to holistic interventions of the mind and body. She now works in a hospital setting and does consulting in wellness and patient focused needs that drive quality and intervention to improve patients getting the best information in their care.

She received an ASN and BSN from Gwynedd-Mercy University in Gwynedd-Valley, Pennsylvania, and an MSN, MBA from the University of Pennsylvania, in Philadelphia PA. She is currently beginning work on her PhD. A wellness guru, she built a career early on in fitness and nutrition driving healthy exercise and lifestyle into the lives of many until her nursing career took the forefront. She is a wife and mother of three wonderful boys. Patti has lived in a variety of places in the USA and has developed a network of collaborative physicians, practitioners, and wellness colleagues.

Contact information : Pattig3fl@icloud.com, fitscriptswellness@gmail.com or www.frozenshoulderhealing.com for further information, or consulting.

ACKNOWLEDGEMENTS

To the wonderful doctors and practitioners who took amazing care helping me diagnose, treat, and heal with stem cell therapy:

The Center for Regenerative Medicine Team (Dr. Farshchian)

1001 NE 125th St, North Miami, FL 33161

www.arthritisusa.net

Dynamic Stem Cell Therapy

2551 N. Green Valley Pkwy., Unit 305 C, Henderson, NV 89014

Stemcellpowernow.com

I am extremely grateful, as they have expertise and empathy to nurture, treat, and guide so that I could heal physically and emotionally with such a devastating enigma of an illness/diseased joint not once, but twice in a lifetime. Through their treatment, and guidance, and my clinical and wellness background, I was able to surpass and overcome the obstacle of this horrible condition.

My Facebook Page:

Frozen Shoulder Wellness & Holistic Alternatives

Consultation & Coaching via Facebook scheduling or email me

at- fitscriptswellness@gmail.com provide name, contact info, and issue

NOTES

NOTES

Lightning Source UK Ltd.
Milton Keynes UK
UKHW010627060122
396716UK00001B/141